Selected Medical Benefits:

Patient Protection and Affordable Care Act of 2010

Introduction

The Patient Protection and Affordable Care Act of 2010 states that "the Secretary [of Health and Human Services] shall define the essential health benefits" for certain health plans. The Act further instructs the Secretary to "ensure that the scope of the essential health benefits … is equal to the scope of benefits provided under a typical employer plan." The Act requires the Secretary of Labor to "conduct a survey of employer-sponsored coverage to determine the benefits typically covered by employers," and to report the results of the survey to the Secretary of Health and Human Services.

To meet its requirement, the Department of Labor (DOL) first looked to its ongoing survey of benefits—the Bureau of Labor Statistics (BLS) National Compensation Survey (NCS). The NCS, a survey of employers, provides comprehensive data on employment-based health care benefits. Annually, data from this survey are released on the percent of employees offered employment-based health care benefits and the percent of employees who are actually covered by such benefits. Further details on the provisions of those health care plans, including what services are covered and what cost-sharing is required by plan participants, are published periodically. Details on the NCS scope and methods may be found in the Technical Note to this report; more comprehensive information is available in the *BLS Handbook of Methods*, Chapter 8: "National Compensation Measures," at http://www.bls.gov/opub/hom/pdf/homch8.pdf.

While the NCS currently captures data from about 36,000 employers, including those in private industry and State and local government across all industries and all establishment sizes, information on the detailed provisions of employment-based health care benefits is from a representative sample of about 3,900 private sector employers annually. From each of these employers, BLS identifies available health plans and requests copies of written documents describing plan benefits. These documents vary widely: some may be formal Summary Plan Descriptions and provide comprehensive information; others may be short summaries or comparison charts that are much less comprehensive. BLS extracted the detailed plan provisions presented in this report from approximately 3,200 plan documents.

Much of the data available from NCS on detailed provisions of employment-based health benefits are from previously-published survey results, which cover such services as hospital room and board, physician office visits, mental health and substance abuse treatment, dental care, and vision care. Cost-sharing information such as deductibles and copayments comes from the previously-published survey results as well. The data are from two separate survey years; in 2008 data were collected on a wide range of health plan provisions; in 2009 data were collected for a smaller subset of health plan provisions. The complete 2008 results are available at http://www.bls.gov/ncs/ebs/detailedprovisions/2008/ebbl0042.pdf. The complete 2009 results are available at

http://www.bls.gov/ncs/ebs/detailedprovisions/2009/ebbl0045.pdf. This report includes new data extracted from the 2009 plan documents on 12 additional health care services and related cost-sharing details.

Summary of previously published NCS information

Type of plan and overall plan limits

Of those employees covered by an employer health benefits plan, 79 percent received benefits under a fee-for-service arrangement in 2009, where payment wasn't made until services were received. The remaining 21 percent were covered by a health maintenance organization (HMO), generally characterized by a fixed set of benefits provided for a prepaid fee, often with restrictions on available providers. Most of those in fee-for-service plans were in the sub-category of plans known as preferred provider organizations (PPOs), where enrollees are provided medical services at a higher level of reimbursement if they receive care from designated providers.

Fee-for-service plans, including PPOs, generally impose certain cost-sharing features referred to here as overall plan limits, which apply to many or all services received. For example, 93 percent of employees covered by a fee-for-service plan had services subject to a deductible, an amount that must be paid before the plan will begin to pay for services. The median annual deductible for all such plans was $500 per person in 2009, although many plans such as PPOs imposed varying deductibles. When plans specified varying deductibles, the median annual deductible was $1,000 per person for out-of-network care but only $500 per person for in-network care.

Once the deductible is met, fee-for-service plans often pay a portion of additional charges. This portion, known as a coinsurance, is often 80 percent, but again can vary based on where services are received. The median in-network coinsurance was 80 percent while the median out-of-network coinsurance was 60 percent. To guard against unusually high health care costs, fee-for-service plans also frequently identify an out-of-pocket expense maximum. Once the employee's share of services (for example, 20 percent) reaches the out-of-pocket expense maximum, future covered charges are paid at 100 percent. In 2009, the median out-of-pocket expense maximum was $1,900 per individual.

Covered services and cost-sharing

Information on coverage and cost-sharing for roughly two dozen medical, dental, and vision services is captured as part of the ongoing survey. For certain common services, such as hospital room and board, inpatient and outpatient surgery, and physician office visits, nearly everyone who has employment-based health benefits has coverage. Other services are provided less often. For example, in 2008 hospital room and board is covered for 99 percent of plan participants while home health care is covered for about 73 percent of plan participants. In the following section, coverage and cost-sharing information is provided for many of the services included in the survey.

As noted, coverage for hospital room and board charges is nearly universal. Table 1 shows that in HMOs, 29 percent of participants have such charges covered in full, with no required cost sharing. The remaining participants were subject to some limits on coverage, such as a copayment per admission. In fee-for-service plans, 92 percent of covered workers are subject to limits; only 7 percent have charges covered in full. Limits in fee-for-service plans include both overall plan limits, such as deductibles and coinsurances discussed previously, and separate limits imposed on the specific service, such as a copayment per hospital admission. The median copayment per admission was $250 in both fee-for-service plans and HMOs.

Table 1. Hospital Room and Board: Type of coverage, private industry workers, National Compensation Survey, 2008

(All workers participating in medical care plans = 100 percent)

Benefit coverage	All plans	Fee-for-service	Health maintenance organizations
Existence of Coverage			
With coverage	99	99	100
Extent of Coverage [1]			
C overed in full	12	7	29
S ubject to limits	88	92	71
Limits on Coverage			
Median copayment per admission	$250	$250	$250

(1) All data are presented as a percent of workers participating in medical care plans. The sum of individual items under "Extent of Coverage" may not equal the "With coverage" value due to rounding and suppression of data that do not meet publication criteria.

NOTE: F or definitions of terms, see *National Compensation Survey: Glossary of Employee Benefit Terms* , available online at http://www.bls.gov/ncs/ebs/glossary20082009.htm. For standard errors and other information on the 2008 survey, see *National Compensation Survey: Health Plan Provisions in Private Industry in the United States, 2008* , available online at http://www.bls.gov/ncs/ebs/detailedprovisions/2008/ebbl0042.pdf.

Coverage for surgical procedures, whether as an inpatient or an outpatient, was nearly always provided to plan participants. Among fee-for-service plans, coverage was subject to limits for 9 out of 10 participants, while the remainder had charges covered in full. This was true for both inpatient and outpatient surgery. There was a somewhat different coverage pattern for inpatient versus outpatient surgery among HMO participants. Slightly more than half—54 percent—of HMO participants had full coverage for inpatient surgery, with the remainder subject to limits such as copayments. In contrast, one-third of HMO participants had full coverage for outpatient surgery. When plans subjected outpatient surgery to a copayment, the median was $50 per visit in fee-for-service plans and $75 per visit in HMOs.

Table 2 shows that all health care plan participants had coverage for physician office visits and nearly all had to share the cost of coverage. The median copayment for a physician office visit was $20 in a fee-for-service plan and $15 in an HMO.

Table 2. Physician Office Visits: Type of coverage, private industry workers, National Compensation Survey, 2008

(All workers participating in medical care plans = 100 percent)

Benefit coverage	All plans	Fee-for-service	Health maintenance organizations
Existence of Coverage			
With coverage	100	100	100
Extent of Coverage [1]			
C overed in full	3	3	–
S ubject to limits	97	97	98
N ot determinable	–	–	(1)
Limits on Coverage			
Median copayment per visit	$20	$20	$15

(1) All data are presented as a percent of workers participating in medical care plans. The sum of individual items under "Extent of Coverage" may not equal the "With coverage" value due to rounding and suppression of data that do not meet publication criteria.

NOTE: Dashes indicate that no data were reported or that data do not meet publication criteria. For definitions of terms, see *National Compensation Survey: Glossary of Employee Benefit Terms* , available online at http://www.bls.gov/ncs/ebs/glossary20082009.htm. For standard errors and other information on the 2008 survey, see *National Compensation Survey: Health Plan Provisions in Private Industry in the United States, 2008* , available online at http://www.bls.gov/ncs/ebs/detailedprovisions/2008/ebbl0042.pdf.

Health plans frequently provide coverage for alternatives to hospitalization. Coverage in a skilled nursing facility was available to 70 percent of participants; coverage for home health and hospice care was available to 73 and 67 percent of participants, respectively. Often, coverage for such services is available following a hospital visit. Plans may impose a limit on the number of days of coverage. The median day limit for skilled nursing facility coverage was 90 days per admission; the median day limit for home health care was 100 days per year.

The survey also provides limited information on certain preventive care services—80 percent of plan participants had coverage for adult physical exams, 77 percent had coverage for well baby care, and 56 percent had coverage for adult immunizations and inoculations.

Coverage for the cost of outpatient prescription drugs is available to nearly all plan participants; 79 percent of participants had the ability to receive ongoing maintenance drugs through a mail-order program. The median copayment for generic drugs was $10 per prescription; the median copayment for brand-name drugs was $25 per prescription.

Considerable detail is captured on coverage for mental health care and substance abuse treatment, although the data presented here pre-date the implementation of the Mental Health Parity and Addiction Equity Act. Table 3 shows that inpatient mental health care and substance abuse detoxification are available to nearly all plan participants (99 percent and 98 percent, respectively), while inpatient substance abuse rehabilitation is available to 78 percent of participants. Outpatient mental health care services are covered for 85 percent of participants; outpatient substance abuse rehabilitation is covered for 79 percent of participants. Such coverage is nearly always subject to limits, including overall plan limits. There is also frequently a limit imposed on the number of days of mental health and substance abuse coverage; the median limit was 30 days per year.

Table 3. Mental Health and Substance Abuse Treatment: Type of coverage, private industry workers, National Compensation Survey, 2008

(All workers participating in medical care plans = 100 percent)

Benefit coverage	All plans	Fee-for-service	Health maintenance organizations
With Coverage			
Inpatient mental health care	99	99	98
Outpatient mental health care	85	84	87
Inpatient substance abuse detoxification	98	98	98
Inpatient substance abuse rehabilitation	78	80	72
Outpatient substance abuse rehabilitation	79	79	79

NOTE: The data in this table pre-date the implementation of the Mental Health Parity and Addiction Equity Act. For definitions of terms, see *National Compensation Survey: Glossary of Employee Benefit Terms*, available online at http://www.bls.gov/ncs/ebs/glossary20082009.htm. For standard errors and other information on the 2008 survey, see *National Compensation Survey: Health Plan Provisions in Private Industry in the United States, 2008*, available online at http://www.bls.gov/ncs/ebs/detailedprovisions/2008/ebbl0042.pdf.

The survey also provides details on plan provisions for those workers who are covered for dental and vision services through an employment-based plan. Plans typically grouped dental services into categories, such as preventive services (typically exams and cleanings), basic services (typically fillings, dental surgery, periodontal care, and endodontic care), major services (typically crowns and prosthetics), and orthodontia. Cost sharing for dental services typically involved an annual deductible—the median was $50 per person. After meeting the deductible, dental plans often paid a percent of covered services up to a maximum annual benefit. The median percent paid by the plan was 100 percent for preventive services, 80 percent for basic services, and 50 percent for major services and orthodontia. The median annual maximum was $1,500; a separate maximum applicable to orthodontic services also had a median value of $1,500.

Workers who had vision coverage nearly always received benefits for eye exams and glasses; 88 percent had coverage for contact lenses. Cost sharing for vision services was identified in a number of ways, including required copayments, fixed dollar amounts paid by the plan, and percentage discounts on the retail price of eye glasses and contact lenses.

Much of the data available from NCS on detailed provisions of employment-based health benefits are from previously-published survey results, which cover such services as hospital room and board, physician office visits, mental health and substance abuse treatment, dental care, and vision care. Cost-sharing information such as deductibles and copayments comes from the previously-published survey results as well. The data are from two separate survey years; in 2008 data were collected on a wide range of health plan provisions; in 2009 data were collected for a smaller subset of health plan provisions. The complete 2008 results are available at http://www.bls.gov/ncs/ebs/detailedprovisions/2008/ebbl0042.pdf. The complete 2009 results are available at http://www.bls.gov/ncs/ebs/detailedprovisions/2009/ebbl0045.pdf.

New information on 12 additional services

To expand the data available from the existing tabulations of the NCS, the Department of Health and Human Services identified additional services for which information on coverage and cost sharing would be helpful. Before conducting a complete extraction from approximately 3,200 plan documents, NCS staff reviewed a small number of these documents to determine data availability. Unfortunately, this review indicated that it is not possible to produce reliable data for many of the services due to the lack of detail that characterizes many plan documents. Services may or may not be covered when they are not mentioned in plan documents.

Sufficient data were available for 12 additional services: emergency room visits, ambulance services, diabetes care management, kidney dialysis, physical therapy, durable medical equipment, prosthetics, maternity care, infertility treatment, sterilization, gynecological exams and services, and organ and tissue transplantation. It is important to note that these services are only a subset of all the services potentially covered by employment-based health insurance plans.

Additional medical services—coverage and cost sharing

The extent to which each of the 12 selected medical benefits was mentioned in the sampled medical plan documentation varied substantially. For example, emergency room visits were mentioned in documents for 9 in 10 participants, whereas diabetes care management, kidney dialysis, and sterilization were mentioned for only 1 in 4 participants. However, if the plan documentation mentioned the benefit, coverage for that benefit was nearly 100 percent—for 10 of the 12 selected benefits studied. The exceptions were infertility treatment, where 6 in 10 medical plan participants were covered for such treatment, and sterilization, where 9 in 10 were covered.

The following chart shows the proportion of each type of medical benefit that was covered, not covered (excluded), or not mentioned in the medical plan documents.

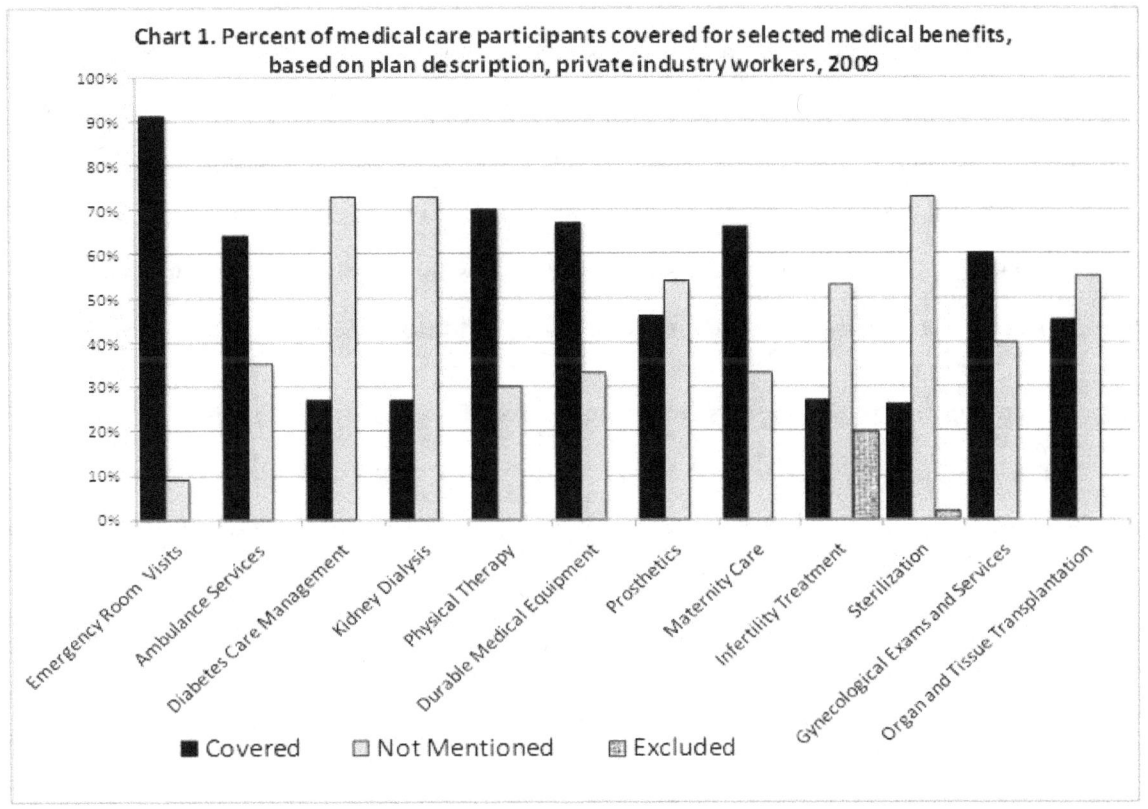

The survey also looked at how medical plans covered these 12 benefits. First, the extent of coverage was examined. Was the benefit covered in full or was coverage limited? Second, the limits applying to each benefit were scrutinized. The survey divided coverage limitations into two main categories: *plan limits* and *separate limits*.

Emergency Room Visits

The term "emergency room visits" was defined as visits to a hospital emergency facility or emergency room due to an accidental injury or a sudden and serious medical condition. Emergency room physician charges were not included under the benefit, but the facility charges were included. When plans differed in coverage between an emergency situation and a non-emergency situation, the coverage for an emergency situation was recorded. Finally, when the type of coverage varied by medical condition, the provisions for life-threatening conditions were recorded, and the provisions for the non-life-threatening conditions were not recorded.

Nine out of ten medical care participants in the survey were covered by emergency care visits, with the remainder of participants in plans where there was no mention of this medical service. Virtually all (89 percent out of 91 percent) of the workers with coverage for emergency room visits had some form of limitation placed on the service; the few remaining workers were provided with full coverage or the extent of their coverage was not mentioned in plan documents.

When limits were present for emergency room visits, it was most common for the workers to be subject to both plan limits and separate limits. Seven out of 10 medical care participants in the survey had their coverage restricted by some form of separate limit. Virtually all of those workers (68 percent out of 70 percent) were subject to a copayment per visit. The median copayment was $100.

A review of plan documents—not of national estimates created from the weighted plan data—revealed that copayments of $50, $75, and $100 were the most prevalent amounts with this restriction. In some instances workers subject to a limit of copayments per visit were also covered at a higher coinsurance rate for this benefit than the overall plan coinsurance. For example, the plan coinsurance was 90 percent while emergency room visits was covered at 100 percent after a $100 copayment.

Incidence of the existence of coverage and the existence of limits for emergency room benefits were similar in fee-for-service plans and health maintenance organizations. However, plan limits were far more likely in fee-for-service plans than in health maintenance organization plans (80 percent and 56 percent, respectively).

Table 4 summarizes the plan provisions for emergency room visits.

Table 4. Emergency Room Visits: Type of coverage, private industry workers, National Compensation Survey, 2009

(All workers participating in medical care plans = 100 percent)

Benefit coverage	All plans	Fee-for-service	Health maintenance organizations
Existence of Coverage			
With coverage	91	90	93
Without coverage	–	–	–
Not mentioned in plan documents	9	10	7
Extent of Coverage [1]			
Covered in full	1	–	–
Subject to limits	89	88	92
Not mentioned in plan documents	1	–	–
Limits on Coverage [2]			
Subject to plan limits	75	80	56
Subject to separate limits	70	64	88
With a copayment per visit	68	62	87
Copayment at 10th percentile	$50	$50	$50
Copayment at 25th percentile	$50	$75	$50
Copayment at 50th percentile (median)	$100	$100	$100
Copayment at 75th percentile	$100	$100	$100
Copayment at 90th percentile	$150	$150	$150
Not mentioned in plan documents	–	–	–

(1) All data are presented as a percent of workers participating in medical care plans. The sum of individual items under "Extent of Coverage" may not equal the "With coverage" value due to rounding and suppression of data that do not meet publication criteria.

(2) All data in the unshaded areas are presented as a percent of workers participating in medical plans. The sum of individual items under "Limits on Coverage" may not equal the "Subject to limits" value due to rounding, suppression of data that do not meet publication criteria, and the fact that some plans may impose more than one limit.

NOTE: Dashes indicate that no data were reported or that data do not meet publication criteria. For standard errors and definitions of terms, see the Technical Note of this report.

Ambulance Services

The term "ambulance services" was defined as transportation by licensed ambulance services to a hospital or an emergency room. If the plan differentiated provisions by type of transportation, the provisions for ground transportation were reported. When coverage for ambulance services varied by type of medical condition, the provisions for emergencies were recorded and the provisions for non-emergencies were not recorded. Finally, when provisions differed for medically necessary conditions and non-medically necessary conditions, the provisions for medically necessary conditions were recorded.

Just under two-thirds of the medical plan participants in the survey were provided coverage for ambulance services, with just about all the remaining third in plans where there was no reference to the benefit. Fifty-two percent of workers had plans that subjected ambulance services to some type of limit, while 10 percent had full coverage. The few remaining workers covered by ambulance services were in plans where the extent of coverage was not described in plan documents.

When ambulance services were subject to limits, it was most common for the limit to be plan limits—for example, deductible and coinsurance. A review of plan documents—not of national estimates created from the weighted plan data—showed that separate limits for this benefit often came in the form of either a different coinsurance than the plan coinsurance or a copayment per trip, commonly ranging from roughly $25 to $100.

Table 5 summarizes the plan provisions for ambulance services.

Table 5. Ambulance Services: Type of coverage, private industry workers, National Compensation Survey, 2009

(All workers participating in medical care plans = 100 percent)

Benefit coverage	All plans	Fee-for-service	Health maintenance organizations
Existence of Coverage			
With coverage	64	65	62
Without coverage	–	–	–
Not mentioned in plan documents	35	35	38
Extent of Coverage [1]			
Covered in full	10	7	–
Subject to limits	52	56	38
Not mentioned in plan documents	2	2	–
Limits on Coverage [2]			
Subject to plan limits	49	54	30
Subject to separate limits	13	10	22
Not mentioned in plan documents	1	1	–

(1) All data are presented as a percent of workers participating in medical care plans. The sum of individual items under "Extent of Coverage" may not equal the "With coverage" value due to rounding and suppression of data that do not meet publication criteria.

(2) All data are presented as a percent of workers participating in medical plans. The sum of individual items under "Limits on Coverage" may not equal the "Subject to limits" value due to rounding, suppression of data that do not meet publication criteria, and the fact that some plans may impose more than one limit.

NOTE: Because of rounding, sums of individual items may not equal totals. Dashes indicate that no data were reported or that data do not meet publication criteria. For standard errors and definitions of terms, see the Technical Note of this report.

Diabetes Care Management

Diabetes care management is the service of educating patients about how to manage this type of illness. For the purpose of this study, coverage for insulin and other diabetic supplies (for example, test strips and needles) was not included under this benefit, since coverage of these items is usually included under a prescription drug plan benefit. If insulin and other supplies were the only benefits described in the plan document, then coverage for diabetes care management was tabulated as "not mentioned." Diabetes care was sometimes included under the general heading of nutritional counseling. Though nutritional counseling in and of itself was not enough to be considered diabetes care, occasionally the general category of nutritional counseling listed diabetes as one of the areas a nutritionist would address. When this situation occurred, diabetes care was recorded as "covered."

As shown in table 6, diabetes care management was one of the least mentioned benefits in the plan documents, with 73 percent of the medical care participants in plans that did not mention the benefit. Nearly all of the remaining 27 percent of medical care participants were in plans in which some form of coverage for diabetes care was provided.

Eighty-three percent of participants in health maintenance organizations had plans that did not mention diabetes care compared to 70 percent of participants with fee-for-service plans. However, for those participants with either type of plan, if diabetes care was mentioned in the plan documents, they almost always had coverage.

Because diabetes care was mentioned in so few documents, information on the extent of coverage did not meet publication standards. (See Technical Note.)

Table 6. Diabetes Care Management: Type of coverage, private industry workers, National Compensation Survey, 2009

(All workers participating in medical care plans = 100 percent)

Benefit coverage	All plans	Fee-for-service	Health maintenance organizations
Existence of Coverage			
With coverage	27	30	17
Without coverage	–	–	–
Not mentioned in plan documents	73	70	83

NOTE: Dashes indicate that no data were reported or that data do not meet publication criteria. For standard errors and definitions of terms, see the Technical Note of this report.

Kidney Dialysis

Kidney dialysis, also called renal dialysis or hemodialysis, is the treatment of an acute or chronic kidney ailment by dialysis methods. Kidney dialysis can take place in a variety of locations, including hospitals, doctors' offices, and outpatient centers. Plan coverage of home dialysis equipment did not meet the survey definition of kidney dialysis.

As can be seen in table 7, kidney dialysis was mentioned in plan documents for about 1 in 4 medical plan participants. In plans in which this benefit was mentioned, nearly all participants were covered for dialysis treatment.

Because kidney dialysis was mentioned in so few documents, information on the extent of coverage did not meet publication standards. (See Technical Note.)

Table 7. Kidney Dialysis: Type of coverage, private industry workers, National Compensation Survey, 2009

(All workers participating in medical care plans = 100 percent)

Benefit coverage	All plans	Fee-for-service	Health maintenance organizations
Existence of Coverage			
With coverage	27	30	19
Without coverage	–	–	–
Not mentioned in plan documents	73	70	81

NOTE: Dashes indicate that no data were reported or that data do not meet publication criteria. For standard errors and definitions of terms, see the Technical Note of this report.

Physical Therapy

Physical therapy was defined as services to restore natural movement to the body, relieve pain, and prevent further injury. Physical therapy can occur in several settings, such as doctors' offices, outpatient hospital departments, inpatient facilities, therapy centers, patients' homes, and nursing facilities. For this survey, provisions for hospital inpatient facilities were not recorded. If plan provisions differed for other locations, the most generous provision (that is, the provision with the least cost to the patient) was recorded.

Plan documents often mentioned physical therapy along with speech therapy and occupational therapy, and sometimes separate limits such as the number of visits covered per year applied to the combination of physical, occupational, and speech therapy. In these cases, the limit was recorded as applicable to physical therapy. For example, if a plan document stated that there was a limit of 60 visits per year for all three types of therapy combined, the 60 visit limit was reported for physical therapy.

Physical therapy was mentioned in plan documents for 7 in 10 medical plan participants. In plans in which this benefit was mentioned, nearly all plan participants were covered.

Nearly all covered participants were subject to limits, most commonly to both plan limits and separate limits for physical therapy. About half the participants subject to separate limits (29 percent out of 55 percent) were required to make a copayment per visit or therapy session. Copayments generally ranged from $10 to $40, and the median was $20.

About 1 in 3 participants (22 percent out of 69 percent with physical therapy coverage) in fee-for-service plans was required to make copayments, while the large majority of health maintenance organization participants (55 percent out of 72 percent that were covered) had a copayment requirement. But the copayment amounts themselves were similar between the two types of plans.

A review of plan documents—not of national estimates created from the weighted plan data—revealed that many plans covering physical therapy limited the number of days or visits paid for per year. Common annual limits were 20, 30, or 60 days or visits. Less frequently observed were day or visit limits per illness or condition or maximum dollar amounts payable per year.

Table 8 summarizes the plan provisions for physical therapy.

Table 8. Physical Therapy: Type of coverage, private industry workers, National Compensation Survey, 2009

(All workers participating in medical care plans = 100 percent)

Benefit coverage	All plans	Fee-for-service	Health maintenance organizations
Existence of Coverage			
With coverage	70	69	72
Without coverage	–	–	–
Not mentioned in plan documents	30	31	28
Extent of Coverage [1]			
Covered in full	–	–	–
Subject to limits	68	68	69
Not mentioned in plan documents	–	–	–
Limits on Coverage [2]			
Subject to plan limits	56	59	43
Subject to separate limits	55	51	67
With a copayment per visit	29	22	55
Copayment at 10th percentile	$10	$15	$10
Copayment at 25th percentile	$15	$20	$15
Copayment at 50th percentile (median)	$20	$20	$20
Copayment at 75th percentile	$30	$30	$30
Copayment at 90th percentile	$40	$35	$40
Not mentioned in plan documents	–	1	–

(1) All data are presented as a percent of workers participating in medical care plans. The sum of individual items under "Extent of Coverage" may not equal the "With coverage" value due to rounding and suppression of data that do not meet publication criteria.

(2) All data in unshaded areas are presented as a percent of workers participating in medical plans. The sum of individual items under "Limits on Coverage" may not equal the "Subject to limits" value due to rounding, suppression of data that do not meet publication criteria, and the fact that some plans may impose more than one limit.

NOTE: Dashes indicate that no data were reported or that data do not meet publication criteria. For standard errors and definitions of terms, see the Technical Note of this report.

Durable Medical Equipment

This benefit was defined as the purchase or rental of equipment or therapeutic supplies to treat medical conditions or improve physical mobility. Examples include oxygen tents, wheelchairs, crutches, canes, walkers, circulatory aids, glucose monitors, cervical collars, and special therapeutic shoes. Provisions for durable medical equipment were described in plan documents for 2 out of 3 medical plan participants. In nearly all plans that mentioned durable medical equipment, participants were covered for the purchase or rental of the equipment.

Most covered participants were subject to coverage limits. Overall, about 3 in 4 were subject to plan limits (51 percent out of 67 percent of participants with durable medical equipment coverage). About 1 in 3 had separate limits (24 percent out of 67 percent). For participants in fee-for-service plans, the limits were most often overall plan limits only, whereas health maintenance organization participants often had separate as well as plan limits.

A review of plan documents—not of national estimates created from the weighted plan data—revealed that the most commonly observed separate limits were dollar maximums per year on the amount of durable medical equipment that the plan would pay. Limits of $2,500 or $5,000 per year were the commonly observed maximums. Other types of dollar limits, such as lifetime dollar maximums and dollar maximums per item of equipment, were much less common. Copayments were rarely imposed.

Table 9 summarizes the plan provisions for durable medical equipment.

Table 9. Durable Medical Equipment: Type of coverage, private industry workers, National Compensation Survey, 2009

(All workers participating in medical care plans = 100 percent)

Benefit coverage	All plans	Fee-for-service	Health maintenance organizations
Existence of Coverage			
With coverage	67	66	67
Without coverage	–	–	–
Not mentioned in plan documents	33	33	33
Extent of Coverage [(1)]			
Covered in full	7	4	–
Subject to limits	57	61	45
Not mentioned in plan documents	2	2	–
Limits on Coverage [(2)]			
Subject to plan limits	51	56	32
Subject to separate limits	24	21	36
Not mentioned in plan documents	2	3	–

(1) All data are presented as a percent of workers participating in medical care plans. The sum of individual items under "Extent of Coverage" may not equal the "With coverage" value due to rounding and suppression of data that do not meet publication criteria.

(2) All data are presented as a percent of workers participating in medical plans. The sum of individual items under "Limits on Coverage" may not equal the "Subject to limits" value due to rounding, suppression of data that do not meet publication criteria, and the fact that some plans may impose more than one limit.

NOTE: Because of rounding, sums of individual items may not equal totals. Dashes indicate that no data were reported or that data do not meet publication criteria. For standard errors and definitions of terms, see the Technical Note of this report.

Prosthetics

Prosthetics, or prostheses, were defined as artificial limbs or replacement devices necessitated by loss or impairment of part of the body. Provisions for prosthetics were mentioned in plan documents for 46 percent of the medical plan participants. When mentioned, prosthetics were nearly always covered by the plan.

Most covered participants were subject to limits, with 44 percent out of 49 percent of covered fee-for-service plan participants subject to limits. Out of 35 percent of health maintenance organization participants covered for prosthetics, 21 percent were subject to limits. Participants in fee-for-service plans were more likely to be subject to plan limits than separate limits (41 compared to 11 percent, respectively), whereas health maintenance organization participants were equally as likely to have separate limits as plan limits (14 percent, each).

A review of plan documents—not of national estimates created from the weighted plan data—showed that, among the plans with separate limits for prosthetics, the most common limits were annual dollar ceilings on plan payments. As with durable medical equipment, dollar caps of $2,500 and $5,000 were the most often seen. Lifetime dollar maximums were uncommon, as were other types of dollar limits such as those imposed per item. Copayments were infrequently observed.

Plan documents sometimes mentioned orthotics when describing the coverage of prosthetics. Orthotics are commonly defined as supplies or equipment that support or correct the function of a limb or torso. But coverage of orthotics alone did not meet the survey definition of prosthetics. Sometimes separate limits such as annual dollar maximums applied to both prosthetics and orthotics. In these cases, the limits were recorded for prosthetics. For example, a plan will pay a maximum of $5,000 per year for prosthetics and orthotics combined. For this plan, the $5,000 limit would be recorded for prosthetics.

Table 10 summarizes the plan provisions for prosthetics.

Table 10. Prosthetics: Type of coverage, private industry workers, National Compensation Survey, 2009

(All workers participating in medical care plans = 100 percent)

Benefit coverage	All plans	Fee-for-service	Health maintenance organizations
Existence of Coverage			
With coverage	46	49	35
Without coverage	–	–	–
Not mentioned in plan documents	54	51	65
Extent of Coverage [(1)]			
Covered in full	5	–	–
Subject to limits	39	44	21
Not mentioned in plan documents	2	–	–
Limits on Coverage [(2)]			
Subject to plan limits	35	41	14
Subject to separate limits	12	11	14
Not mentioned in plan documents	2	2	–

(1) All data are presented as a percent of workers participating in medical care plans. The sum of individual items under "Extent of Coverage" may not equal the "With coverage" value due to rounding and suppression of data that do not meet publication criteria.

(2) All data are presented as a percent of workers participating in medical plans. The sum of individual items under "Limits on Coverage" may not equal the "Subject to limits" value due to rounding, suppression of data that do not meet publication criteria, and the fact that some plans may impose more than one limit.

NOTE: Dashes indicate that no data were reported or that data do not meet publication criteria. For standard errors and definitions of terms, see the Technical Note of this report.

Maternity Care

Maternity care can refer to a variety of services. It may mean care throughout the woman's pregnancy or it may mean care during the time spent in the hospital just before and after giving birth. For the purpose of this study, maternity care was defined as the medical coverage throughout the woman's pregnancy; it included such diagnostic testing as ultrasounds and fetal monitor procedures.

Plan documents often separated maternity care into three stages: prenatal, delivery, and postnatal. The stages included different types of services; in some plans the stages were covered differently. Hospitalization for delivery was often covered the same as regular inpatient care; prenatal care was sometimes subject to a copayment per office visit or per pregnancy. When there were differences in coverage, provisions for prenatal care were reported. In addition, when coverage varied by the type of doctor performing the treatment, the copayment rate for a specialist was reported rather than the copayment rate for a primary care physician.

Two-thirds of the medical care participants in the survey were covered by maternity care, with almost all of the remaining third in plans in which the benefit was not mentioned. The vast majority of workers with coverage were subject to some type of limitation (58 percent out of 66 percent with coverage). A small group of workers were in plans where maternity care was covered in full.

Maternity care was most likely to be subject to either plan limits or both separate limits and plan limits. When there were separate limits on maternity care, it was usually in the form of a copayment per visit. The median copayment was $20, with amounts generally ranging from $10 to $40 per visit. Copayments per visit for maternity care applied either throughout the pregnancy or for a limited number of visits.

A review of plan documents—not of national estimates created from the weighted plan data—showed that if the plan required copayments per visit *for a limited number of visits,* the plan almost always required the copayment only the initial visit. Another separate limit for maternity care less frequently found in plan documents was a higher coinsurance rate than the plan coinsurance rate.

The percentage of medical care participants covered by fee-for-service and health maintenance organization plans for maternity care was identical, each at 66 percent. However, there were differences in the extent of coverage between these two types of plans. It was far more likely for health maintenance organizations to cover maternity care in full than fee-for-service plans (16 percent and 4 percent, respectively). Fee-for-service plans were more likely to cover maternity care subject to plan limits than health maintenance organizations (55 percent and 32 percent, respectively).

Table 11 summarizes the plan provisions for maternity care.

Table 11. Maternity Care: Type of coverage, private industry workers, National Compensation Survey, 2009

(All workers participating in medical care plans = 100 percent)

Benefit coverage	All plans	Fee-for-service	Health maintenance organizations
Existence of Coverage			
With coverage	66	66	66
Without coverage	–	–	–
Not mentioned in plan documents	33	33	34
Extent of Coverage [1]			
Covered in full	6	4	16
Subject to limits	58	61	49
Not mentioned in plan documents	2	2	1
Limits on Coverage [2]			
Subject to plan limits	50	55	32
Subject to separate limits	36	34	45
With a copayment per visit	30	27	41
Copayment at 10th percentile	$10	$15	$10
Copayment at 25th percentile	$15	$20	$15
Copayment at 50th percentile (median)	$20	$20	$20
Copayment at 75th percentile	$30	$30	$30
Copayment at 90th percentile	$40	$40	$40
Not mentioned in plan documents	2	2	–

(1) All data are presented as a percent of workers participating in medical care plans. The sum of individual items under "Extent of Coverage" may not equal the "With coverage" value due to rounding and suppression of data that do not meet publication criteria.

(2) All data in unshaded areas are presented as a percent of workers participating in medical plans. The sum of individual items under "Limits on Coverage" may not equal the "Subject to limits" value due to rounding, suppression of data that do not meet publication criteria, and the fact that some plans may impose more than one limit.

NOTE: Because of rounding, sums of individual items may not equal totals. Dashes indicate that no data were reported or that data do not meet publication criteria. For standard errors and definitions of terms, see the Technical Note of this report.

Infertility Treatment

Infertility treatments include services to diagnose and treat the causes of infertility and may include many different methods for assisted reproduction such as artificial insemination, ovulation induction, in-vitro fertilization, and other advanced reproductive technology. Infertility treatment was not considered "covered" in plans that covered only diagnosis—and not treatment.

Infertility treatment can take place in a variety of settings, in large part because treatment can involve several stages. Some plans only pay for treatment of the underlying conditions causing infertility. Other plans pay for various methods of promoting pregnancy, which can require treatment ranging from consultations, examinations, and procedures accomplished during physician's office visits to inpatient surgery.

Plan coverage provisions were sometimes simple to summarize when the provisions were directly comparable; for example, a copayment for treatment at a doctor's office and a copayment for treatment at a hospital outpatient facility. At the other extreme, the coverage provisions could include a mix of plan and separate limits for different treatment settings, so that the recording of plan provisions for the entire benefit was complex. If coverage for infertility services varied by location, the provisions for "outpatient settings" were recorded. Also, coinsurance rates for infertility services that differed from the overall plan coinsurance rate were recorded. Other separate limits, such as copayments for physician office visits and maximum dollar limits for infertility services, were recorded but not weighted to create national estimates.

Infertility treatment was mentioned in the plan documents for 47 percent of medical plan participants. Almost 3 in 5 participants were covered (27 percent out of 47 percent); the remaining 2 in 5 participants (20 percent out of 47 percent) were specifically excluded from coverage. Covered services were almost always subject to plan or separate limits.

Participants in health maintenance organization plans that mentioned infertility treatment more often had coverage than those in fee-for-service plans (32 percent out of 44 percent that mentioned the benefit compared to 26 percent out of 48 percent, respectively). However, nearly all covered participants had limits on this benefit. For example, 30 percent out of 32 percent of participants in health maintenance organizations, and 25 percent out of 26 percent of participants in fee-for-service plans, had limits. Coverage for participants *with limits* more frequently included separate limits in health maintenance organization plans (28 percent out of 30 percent with limits) compared with fee-for-service plans (17 percent out of 25 percent with limits). The reverse was true for plan limits (16 percent out of 30 percent and 21 percent out of 25 percent, respectively).

Separate limits for infertility treatments were varied. Separate coinsurance rates for infertility services were observed in plans covering about 1 in 4 participants with separate limits for infertility treatments (5 percent out of 19 percent). The coinsurance rate most often seen was 50 percent, although the 50-percent coinsurance rate tabulated for the 75th percentile, has a large standard error (17.5 percent). A review of plan documents—not of national estimates created from the weighted plan data—revealed that separate limits commonly included copayments for physician office visits and maximum dollar limits per year or per lifetime for infertility treatment coverage.

Table 12 summarizes the plan provisions for infertility treatment.

Table 12. Infertility Treatment: Type of coverage, private industry workers, National Compensation Survey, 2009

(All workers participating in medical care plans = 100 percent)

Benefit coverage	All plans	Fee-for-service	Health maintenance organizations
Existence of Coverage			
With coverage	27	26	32
Without coverage	20	22	12
Not mentioned in plan documents	53	52	56
Extent of Coverage [(1)]			
Covered in full	[(2)]	–	[(2)]
Subject to limits	26	25	30
Not mentioned in plan documents	1	–	1
Limits on Coverage [(3)]			
Subject to plan limits	20	21	16
Subject to separate limits	19	17	28
With a coinsurance per visit	5	2	15
Coinsurance at 10th percentile	50	50	50
Coinsurance at 25th percentile	50	50	50
Coinsurance at 50th percentile (median)	50	50	50
Coinsurance at 75th percentile	50	90	50
Coinsurance at 90th percentile	90	100	70
Not mentioned in plan documents	2	1	–

(1) All data are presented as a percent of workers participating in medical care plans. The sum of individual items under "Extent of Coverage" may not equal the "With coverage" value due to rounding and suppression of data that do not meet publication criteria.

(2) Less than 0.5 percent.

(3) All data in unshaded areas are presented as a percent of workers participating in medical plans. The sum of individual items under "Limits on Coverage" may not equal the "Subject to limits" value due to rounding, suppression of data that do not meet publication criteria, and the fact that some plans may impose more than one limit.

NOTE: Dashes indicate that no data were reported or that data do not meet publication criteria. For standard errors and definitions of terms, see the Technical Note of this report.

Sterilization

Sterilization includes surgical procedures for men and women to prevent future pregnancies, commonly vasectomy for men and tubal ligation for women. Sterilization reversal was not included as part of this benefit. Sterilization can take place in a variety of treatment settings: physician offices, surgical centers, as well as outpatient and inpatient hospital surgical facilities. Additionally, surgery is often preceded by visits to the surgeon's office for examinations and consultations.

As shown in table 13, sterilization coverage was not mentioned in plan documents for 73 percent of plan participants. When it was mentioned, sterilization was a covered benefit for about 9 in 10 participants (26 percent out of 27 percent of participants in plans that mentioned the benefit).

Because sterilization was mentioned in so few documents, information on the extent of coverage did not meet publication standards. (See Technical Note.)

Table 13. Sterilization: Type of coverage, private industry workers, National Compensation Survey, 2009

(All workers participating in medical care plans = 100 percent)

Benefit coverage	All plans	Fee-for-service	Health maintenance organizations
Existence of Coverage			
With coverage	26	27	20
Without coverage	2	2	1
Not mentioned in plan documents	73	71	79

NOTE: Because of rounding, sums of individual items may not equal totals. For standard errors and definitions of terms, see the Technical Note of this report.

Gynecological Exams and Services

Gynecological exams and services include routine gynecological exams, pelvic examinations and/or Papanicolaou (PAP) tests. Plan documents often called gynecological exams "well woman exams" and "pelvic exams." Gynecological services were considered as "covered" if the plan included coverage for a PAP test or if the plan made any reference to the obstetrical and gynecological medical specialties. Plan references only to "preventive care" and "annual physicals" were not considered gynecological exams and services.

The range of gynecological services and tests represented in this benefit category includes various coverage conditions. Some plan documents described coverage for PAP tests but not for gynecological exams. In these cases, the limits on PAP tests were recorded. Caution should be taken when using the data on separate limits for gynecological exams and services because the limits recorded applied in some cases to all services and in other cases to some of the services.

Sixty percent of participants had coverage for gynecological exams and services; for almost all of the remaining 40 percent of participants, plan documents did not mention these services.

In plans in which gynecological exams and services were mentioned, the services were almost always subject to plan or separate limits. Separate limits were in force for 9 in 10 participants in plans with limits on this service (51 percent out of 56 percent), and for a sizeable majority of them (33 percent out of 51 percent), a copayment was required for physician office visits. Copayments commonly ranged from $15 to $25. Copayments for physician office visits often varied by type of doctor. The copayment rate for a specialist was recorded instead of the copayment rate for a primary care physician (PCP) unless the plan instructed otherwise or indicated that the obstetrician-gynecologist medical specialist was considered a PCP. The copayment estimates for this service represent a mix of PCP and specialist copayment rates.

The plan documents revealed information on other separate limits; however it was not weighted to create national estimates. Other separate limits for gynecological exams and services commonly included a limit on the number of exams per year (one per year was most common), a dollar limit on the covered costs for the exam, and higher coinsurance rates than paid by the plan (100 percent was common).

When plan documents for fee-for-service and health maintenance organization plans mentioned gynecological exams and services, coverage provisions were somewhat similar. If the benefit was mentioned in the plan, both types of plans almost always provided coverage. Regardless of plan type, 9 in 10 of those covered had limits on these services (56 percent out of 60 percent). However, the use of plan limits was far more common in fee-for-service plans (49 percent out of 62 percent) than in health maintenance organizations (28 percent out of 52 percent).

Table 14 summarizes the plan provisions for gynecological exams and services.

Table 14. Gynecological Exams and Services: Type of coverage, private industry workers, National Compensation Survey, 2009

(All workers participating in medical care plans = 100 percent)

Benefit coverage	All plans	Fee-for-service	Health maintenance organizations
Existence of Coverage			
With coverage	60	62	52
Without coverage	–	–	–
Not mentioned in plan documents	40	38	48
Extent of Coverage [1]			
Covered in full	–	–	–
Subject to limits	56	58	47
Not mentioned in plan documents	–	–	–
Limits on Coverage [2]			
Subject to plan limits	44	49	28
Subject to separate limits	51	53	45
With a copayment per visit	33	31	39
Copayment at 10th percentile	$10	–	$10
Copayment at 25th percentile	$15	–	$15
Copayment at 50th percentile (median)	$20	–	$20
Copayment at 75th percentile	$25	–	$30
Copayment at 90th percentile	$35	–	$40
Not mentioned in plan documents	–	–	–

(1) All data are presented as a percent of workers participating in medical care plans. The sum of individual items under "Extent of Coverage" may not equal the "With coverage" value due to rounding and suppression of data that do not meet publication criteria.

(2) All data in unshaded areas are presented as a percent of workers participating in medical plans. The sum of individual items under "Limits on Coverage" may not equal the "Subject to limits" value due to rounding, suppression of data that do not meet publication criteria, and the fact that some plans may impose more than one limit.

NOTE: Dashes indicate that no data were reported or that data do not meet publication criteria. For standard errors and definitions of terms, see the Technical Note of this report.

Organ and Tissue Transplantation

Organ and tissue transplantation are medical procedures by which human organs or tissues are transferred from a donor to a recipient. For this survey, transplantation surgery for a major body organ, such as the kidney, liver, and heart, must not be excluded. Coverage was recorded for the organ or tissue recipient but not for the donor.

Organ and tissue transplantation always involves various stages and various settings. Consultation and diagnosis may occur at a doctor's office or transplantation center. Evaluation typically occurs at a transplantation center. After a suitable organ or suitable tissues have been located and matched to the patient, surgery generally occurs at a hospital or surgical center. The final stages, recovery and follow up examinations, can also occur in different settings. As a result, the survey recorded the coverage provided for the surgical procedure. When organ and tissue transplantation services were covered more generously (that is, at a lower cost to the patient) when performed in a designated transplantation center, these more generous provisions were recorded.

As can be seen in table 15, "organ and tissue transplantation" was mentioned in plan documents for just less than one-half of all participants (45 percent), but in plans in which this benefit was mentioned, nearly all plans provided coverage. In the plans with coverage, limits applied to 7 in 8 participants (39 percent out of 45 percent). The remaining participants were evenly divided (3 percent, each) in plans with full coverage or in plans for which the extent of coverage was not mentioned. When there were limits, plan limits were about twice as prevalent as separate limits (32 percent compared to 17 percent). A review of plan documents—not of national estimates created from the weighted plan data—revealed that the most common forms of separate limits were maximum dollar limits (for each transplantation, or per year or lifetime, or for organ or tissue procurement), higher coinsurance rates (particularly if the transplantation was done in a designated transplantation facility), and copayments for physician office visits.

As noted, fee-for-service and health maintenance organization plans almost always provided coverage for organ and tissue transplantation *when mentioned in plan documents*. However, limits on the coverage differed between these types of plans. For those covered, there was a higher percent of participants in fee-for-service plans subject to limits (44 percent out of 48 percent) than of those in health maintenance organization plans (18 percent out of 31 percent). In fee-for-service plans with limits, plan limits were far more common than separate limits (37 percent compared to 18 percent, respectively). In health maintenance organizations, about equal percentages of participants were covered by plan limits and separate limits (11 percent and 10 percent).

Table 15. Organ and Tissue Transplantation: Type of coverage, private industry workers, National Compensation Survey, 2009

(All workers participating in medical care plans = 100 percent)

Benefit coverage	All plans	Fee-for-service	Health maintenance organizations
Existence of Coverage			
With coverage	45	48	31
W ithout coverage	–	–	–
N ot mentioned in plan documents	55	51	69
Extent of Coverage [(1)]			
C overed in full	3	–	7
S ubject to limits	39	44	18
N ot mentioned in plan documents	3	–	7
Limits on Coverage [(2)]			
S ubject to plan limits	32	37	11
Subject to separate limits	17	18	10
N ot mentioned in plan documents	4	4	–

(1) All data are presented as a percent of workers participating in medical care plans. The sum of individual items under "Extent of Coverage" may not equal the "With coverage" value due to rounding and suppression of data that do not meet publication criteria.

(2) All data are presented as a percent of workers participating in medical plans. The sum of individual items under "Limits on Coverage" may not equal the "Subject to limits" value due to rounding, suppression of data that do not meet publication criteria, and the fact that some plans may impose more than one limit.

NOTE: Because of rounding, sums of individual items may not equal totals. Dashes indicate that no data were reported or that data do not meet publication criteria. For standard errors and definitions of terms, see the Technical Note of this report.

Technical note

The National Compensation Survey (NCS) is a survey of employers that provides comprehensive measures of occupational earnings, employer costs of employee compensation, compensation trends, wages in one geographic area relative to other geographic areas, the incidence of employer-provided benefits among workers, and provisions of employer-provided benefit plans. The NCS surveys workers in private industry establishments, and in State and local government, in the 50 States and the District of Columbia. For the NCS, the term "civilian worker" denotes workers in private industry and workers in State and local government. Establishments with one or more workers are included in the survey. Major exclusions from the survey are workers in Federal and quasi-Federal agencies, military personnel, agricultural workers, workers in private households, the self-employed, volunteers, unpaid workers, individuals receiving long-term disability compensation, and individuals working overseas. The NCS also excludes individuals who set their own pay (for example, proprietors, owners, major stockholders, and partners in unincorporated firms) and family members being paid token wages.

BLS field economists employ a variety of methods to obtain data from NCS survey respondents, including personal visits, mail, telephone, and email. The field economist collects summary plan descriptions or similar plan documents for the health and retirement plans offered by the employer. These documents are analyzed by BLS economists to determine detailed provisions of health and retirement plans. Detailed benefits provisions data are collected from the private industry establishments that are in their initial 14 months in the survey, which, for the NCS, is from May of one year through July of the next year. Annual data are published in the summer of the next year.

Most of the tables in this report indicate the percentage of all employees participating in medical benefits or the percentage covered by a specific provision. The base of each table is indicated by the statement under the title that indicates what subset of workers equals 100 percent. The data appearing in the benefit tables and the chart are estimates representing medical plan participants in private industry. Some tables in this report contain fields with estimates classified as "not determinable." Situations that result in this classification can vary. In detailed provisions of employer-provided health care plans, the "not determinable" classification is used whenever partial information on a particular plan feature is available from the summary plan description. Another situation in which the "not determinable" classification may be used is when workers are participating in plans in which a provision is known to exist, but no information on the specific details of this provision is available.

For the 12 additional medical services studied, some information gleaned from the data entered into the "Remarks" areas of the computer system were used to provide additional insights into the data—specifically on the types of separate limits for the benefit. These insights are based only upon a review of the medical plans analyzed; none of these data have been weighted to create nationally representative estimates for medical plan participants.

A variety of approaches were used to manage the quality of the data captured and estimates produced for this study. Initially, the project analysts were provided with detailed survey procedures and training. Thereafter, they prepared a plan for quality management that included a peer audit to certify each analyst's understanding of survey definitions and procedures, use of data entry system edits to ensure the completeness and logical consistency of the entered data, and queries of the database entries to identify entries that were outside of reasonableness parameters as well as unusual entries. Estimate production included an extensive validation of survey estimates to ensure that estimation methods yielded expected results.

Publication standards were set, as they are for all NCS products, to protect confidentiality of data reported by sampled establishments and maintain a specified level of reliability for published estimates.

Procedures and definitions for extraction of information on 12 additional medical services

Analysts scrutinized plan documents for information on 12 medical benefits that are not studied in the regular BLS survey:

Emergency room visits	Ambulance services	Diabetes care management
Kidney dialysis	Physical therapy	Durable medical equipment
Prosthetics	Maternity care	Infertility treatment
Sterilization	Gynecological exams and services	Organ transplantation

Each of these terms is defined below. The survey used three or four questions to describe how medical care plans covered these 12 benefits.

Question 1: Was the benefit covered?

Analysts answered this question for each medical plan included in the 2009 Selected Medical Benefits Report. There were three answers to this question:

- The benefit was covered by the plan. That is, the plan paid for designated services or goods.
- The benefit was excluded by the plan. That is, the plan explicitly stated that the benefit was not covered.
- The benefit was not mentioned in the plan documents.

Question 2: How was the benefit covered by the plan?

For plans that covered the benefit, analysts answered question 2. There were three answers to choose from:

- The benefit was covered in full. That is, the plan paid 100 percent of eligible costs.
- Coverage was subject to limits. The plan placed restrictions on how much it would pay of eligible costs.
- Information on how the plan covered the benefit was not described in plan documents.

Question 3: What limits applied to the benefit?

For plans that had limits on coverage, analysts answered question 3. There were four answers to choose from:

- ***Plan limits applied***. These are restrictions on coverage that apply to most or all medical benefits in the plan. The ongoing BLS survey currently collects data on these limits.

  - A ***deductible*** is a fixed dollar amount that an insured person must pay during the benefit period—usually a year—before the plan begins to make payments for covered medical services.

- *Coinsurance* is the percentage of covered charges paid by the insurer after the annual deductible, if any, is paid.
- *Maximum out-of-pocket expense* provisions limit the dollar amount an insured is required to pay during a year.
- *Maximum lifetime dollar limits* are ceilings on the amount of covered expenses that the insurer will pay.

- *Separate limits applied.* These are restrictions that apply to an individual benefit, rather than a group of benefits. The most prominent separate limit published in the survey is a *copayment*. A copayment is the fixed dollar amount that an insured person must pay when a service is received before any remaining charges are paid by the plan. For example, emergency room visits are subject to a $100 copayment per visit. Other types of separate limits include annual maximum dollar payments for a particular benefit, coinsurance rates for a benefit that differs from the plan's rate, and limits on the number of visits or treatments.

- *Both plan and separate limits applied.* Many workers participating in medical plans were subject to *both* plan and separate limits for the benefits surveyed.

- *Limits unknown.* Information on how limits applied to the benefit was not described in plan documents.

Question 4: What were the separate limits?

For several of the benefits, a fourth question was asked for plans that imposed separate limits on coverage. There were several answers to choose from:

- Was there a copayment per visit? How much was the copayment?
- Was there a copayment per visit and another kind of separate limit? How much was the copayment? What was the other separate limit?
- If there was no copayment required, was there another kind of separate limit? What was the other separate limit?

Copayments for Some Benefits. The dollar amount of copayments was entered into an answer box for several benefits (emergency room visits, diabetes care management, kidney dialysis, physical therapy, durable medical equipment, maternity care, and gynecological exams and services). For one of the benefits studied, infertility treatment, information was asked about whether a separate coinsurance rate applied, rather than a copayment. This was a coinsurance rate that differed from the overall plan rate.

To yield additional insights into these 12 selected medical benefits, information on the type of medical plan from the regular survey was combined with the data from this special survey. Information was published for two broad types of medical plan: *fee-for-service* plans and *health maintenance organization* plans. The former plan finances, but does not deliver, health care services; employers pay premiums to a private insurance carrier to provide a specific set of health benefits. The latter plan assumes both the financial risk associated with providing comprehensive medical services and the responsibility for delivering health care in a particular geographic area, usually in return for a fixed prepaid fee from its members.

General Instructions on Plan and Separate Limits

Analysts used the following instructions in recording information on plan and separate limits.

Plan Limits

Being subject to plan limits (overall limits) means that a benefit:

a) Accrues toward the out-of-pocket maximum;
b) Accrues toward a lifetime maximum, if there is one;
c) Is subject to the deductible; and/or
d) Is covered at the same coinsurance as the coinsurance for the majority of services.

Report that the benefit is subject to plan limits if one or more of these conditions are met.

Separate Limits

Often these separate limits come in the form of a copayment, though it may sometimes be a coinsurance that is different from the overall plan coinsurance, a dollar maximum, or a day/visit limit.

Example: The overall plan deductible, coinsurance, and lifetime maximum benefit apply to physical therapy services. In addition, the plan pays for a maximum of 30 visits or treatments per year. The limit on visits is a separate limit.

Note that a separate limit may be a more generous (lower cost to patient) benefit than the plan limit.

Report as separate limits cases where a different *overall* limit is imposed. The only cases of this occurring are if a different coinsurance rate applies to the benefit. If an overall limit is lifted, rather than imposed, do not report this as a separate limit.

Example: If the plan deductible does not apply to a particular benefit, or if expenses incurred for a benefit do not count towards the out-of-pocket maximum, do not consider these cases as constituting a separate limit.

Some benefits that cover a variety of goods or services (such as organ transplants or durable medical equipment) are subject to a number of "inner limits," limits that apply to some, but not all, of the goods and services covered. Report only limits that apply to the entire benefit, such as an annual maximum for the benefit (example, $1,500 a year for durable medical equipment). Another example would be the imposition of a deductible specific to the benefit.

Documentation Exception: If a dollar limit applies to a specific organ, such as a $50,000 maximum for a kidney transplant, record the limit in Remarks. Note that a distinction is made between a dollar limit on what the plan will pay for any single organ versus a dollar limit on a specific, designated organ. The former applies to the entire benefit, since an organ transplant requires an organ. The latter, however, applies only to one of the major organs covered by the benefit.

For most of the 12 benefits, report a dollar amount if a copayment is listed in the plan document. Besides dollar copayments, if there is an additional separate limit either in place of or in addition to a copayment, the analyst must indicate that an "other separate limit" exists and describe the limit in the Remarks area (Note: For infertility treatment, coinsurance rates rather than copayments are coded.)

Several other general guidelines to remember when reporting separate limits:

- If several different copayments are present for a particular benefit, code for the most generous (i.e., the lowest) copayment, unless the guidance for that benefit specifies otherwise. (See special copayment or coinsurance instructions for: emergency room visits, maternity care, infertility services, and gynecological exams.)

- If coinsurances or copayments differ between in and out-of-network, report for in-network services only. (Some plans provide coverage through a network of participating health care providers. Enrollees may receive coverage outside the network, but at higher costs.)

- In some plans, the maternity care copayment only applies to the first visit, with the rest of the visits over the course of the woman's pregnancy covered with no copayment. In these cases, report the one-time dollar copayment in the copayment box, and explain in Remarks that it is a one-time copayment.

- Also use this procedure for other benefits if one-time copayments apply.

Specific Instructions for Each of the 12 Benefits

Data analysts used a uniform set of instructions (survey procedures) to answer the 4 questions describing how the benefits were covered in each of the medical plans studied. These instructions are summarized below.

Emergency Room Visits

Definition

This benefit includes visits to a hospital emergency facility or emergency room due to accidental injury or a sudden and serious medical condition. Emergency room visits include the facility charges but not the physician charges.

Synonyms: Emergency care, emergency room care, emergency services, and emergency department visits. Urgent care, however, is not the same thing as emergency care, and should not be collected.

Data Analysis Instructions

Occasionally plans will differentiate between coverage for emergency situations and non-emergency situations. For this survey, report the provisions for emergency situations. If the plan does not differentiate between emergency and non-emergency cases, assume that the coverage limits are for emergency services.

Other guidelines are: (a) Code for life-threatening conditions if coverage varies by condition. (b) If coverage varies by other factors, code for the most generous copayment (least cost to the patient); but describe the provision in Remarks.

Instructions on Separate Limits

Report dollar copayment amounts in the box provided. A common limit for emergency room visits is a copayment (also called an access fee), which most commonly is waived if the patient is admitted to the hospital following a stay in the emergency room. Report the dollar copayment limit regardless of whether the plan stipulates that it be waived. Also indicate if emergency room visits are covered at a different coinsurance than other services in the plan, because this is a type of separate limit. All other separate limits should be described in Remarks.

One way that limits are sometimes described for emergency room visits is as a benefit-specific deductible, rather than a copayment. For example, a plan may say that the overall plan coinsurance applies for emergency room visits, but first a $50 emergency room deductible must be met. Treat the deductible as a copayment, and report $50 as the separate limit for this benefit.

Ambulance Services

Definition

This benefit is transportation via licensed ambulance service to a hospital or emergency room.

Synonym: Emergency transportation.

Data Analysis Instructions

If the plan differentiates between ambulance coverage for emergency situations and non-emergency situations, capture only the provisions for emergency situations. If the plan does not differentiate between emergency and non-emergency, consider that the coverage limits are for emergency services.

Similarly, many plans only pay for ambulance services in "medically necessary" situations. If limits vary for medically necessary versus not medically necessary situation, report only for medically necessary situations.

Plans sometimes specify that ground, air, and water ambulance services are all covered. Usually the limits for these different types of ambulances are the same. In the event that the limits differ for these three types, report the limits for ground ambulance services only.

Instructions on Separate Limit:

Analysts will report for whether there are any separate limits for ambulance services, but will not be prompted to enter a specific copayment. However, all separate limits should be described in Remarks.

Diabetes Care Management

Definition

Diabetes care or diabetes care management is defined as the service of educating patients about how to manage their diabetes. Coverage for insulin and other diabetes supplies (test strips, lancets, needles, etc.) are not included in this benefit, since supplies and devices are usually included in prescription drug plans. Therefore, if the only mention is for insulin or other supplies, report that diabetes care management is not mentioned.

If diabetes care is mentioned without a description of the type of services covered, assume that some training and education is included.

Though nutritional counseling alone is not synonymous with diabetes care, sometimes the description of nutritional counseling lists diabetes as one of the areas a nutritionist will address.

Synonyms: Diabetes management, diabetes self-management, diabetes education, training, or consultation, and diabetes treatment.

Instructions on Separate Limits

Report the dollar amount of copayments per visit. All other separate limits should be described in Remarks.

Example: A plan document describes diabetes care as follows

Diabetes Care Benefits:

- Devices, equipment, and supplies covered at 20 percent coinsurance
- Diabetes self-management training and education: $15 per visit

Action: In this example, the analyst should code that there are separate limits for this benefit and record the $15 copayment.

Kidney Dialysis

Definition

Kidney dialysis is defined as the treatment of an acute or chronic kidney ailment by dialysis methods. Dialysis is usually considered an outpatient service. Coverage of home dialysis equipment does not meet our criteria, because we are interested in the coverage for hospital, office visits, or outpatient centers. Home dialysis equipment is usually considered a type of durable medical equipment.

Synonyms: Renal dialysis, hemodialysis, and dialysis.

Data Analysis Instructions

If dialysis coverage varies by location (such as office visit versus hospital outpatient facility), report the most generous provision (the one resulting in lowest cost to the patient), but describe the other provisions in Remarks.

Instructions on Separate Limits

Report dollar copayment limits. Also, indicate other limits, such as a dollar maximum (either per lifetime or per benefit period) for benefits related to kidney disease or a different coinsurance rate in Remarks.

Example: The plan states that kidney dialysis varies depending upon where treatment occurs: (1) $30 copayment per office visit or (2) $100 copayment in the outpatient facility of the hospital.

Action: Report the copayment for office visits as the most generous (least cost to the patient) benefit, but describe the other provisions in Remarks.

Physical Therapy

Definition

Physical therapy is a benefit that covers services to restore movement, relieve pain, and prevent further injury.

Synonyms: Physical medicine and rehabilitation benefits.

Data Analysis Instructions

Report only the limits for office visits, home visits, outpatient hospital departments, and other outpatient facilities. If the copayment is not the same for these four locations, report the lowest copayment. Coverage for inpatient rehabilitation facilities is out of scope for this survey. These facilities, including skilled nursing facilities and inpatient rehabilitation units of hospitals, usually have higher copayments.

Instructions on Separate Limits

Report dollar copayment amounts. Describe other limits, such as the number of physical therapy visits/treatments per year or a benefit maximum (e.g., $5,000 for physical therapy per benefit period) in Remarks.

Physical therapy is also often grouped with occupational and speech therapy, with the same limits listed for all three therapies. If therapy provisions are stated separately for occupational, speech, and physical therapy, report the provision for physical therapy alone.

Example: The plan states that there is a combined limit of 60 visits per year for physical, occupational, and speech therapy.

Action: Report the 60 visits as a separate limit for physical therapy.

Example: The plan states occupational therapy provisions separately from physical therapy.

Action: Report for physical therapy alone.

Durable Medical Equipment

Definition

Durable medical equipment (DME) usually includes the rental or purchase of equipment or therapeutic supplies to treat medical conditions or improve physical mobility. Examples of such equipment are oxygen tents, wheelchairs, crutches, canes, walkers, circulatory aids, glucose monitors, cervical collars, and special therapeutic shoes. Generally the equipment must be prescribed by a physician in order to be covered by the plan.

Instructions on Separate Limits

Report the dollar copayment per item. Describe other separate limits such as benefit maximums per calendar year in Remarks.

If a separate limit is listed for rental of equipment versus repair or replacement of equipment, code for rental only.

Prosthetics

Definition

Prosthetics are defined as artificial limbs necessitated by the loss or impairment of part of the body. Generally prosthetics are covered only to the extent that the device restores the basic function lost as a result of disease or accidental injury, and they must be prescribed by a physician. Orthotics, which are defined as supplies and equipment to support or correct the function of a limb or torso, are sometimes combined with coverage for prosthetics, but coverage for orthotics alone does not meet the survey definition of prosthetics. "Corrective appliances" is used in some plans as a synonym for prosthetics but is defined as orthotics in other plans; this study considers corrective appliances to be prosthetics only the when plan documents define it as prosthetics.

Synonyms: Prosthetic devices, prostheses, durable medical equipment including prosthetics, and external prosthetic appliances.

Instructions on Separate Limits

Analysts will report for whether there are any separate limits for prosthetics, but will not be prompted to enter a specific copayment. However, all separate limits should be described in Remarks.

Example: *The plan covers prosthetics and orthotics. It states that an annual dollar limit applies to prosthetics and orthotics.*

Action: Report the dollar maximum as applying to prosthetics.

Maternity Care

Definition

Maternity care may refer to a number of different services. Sometimes the term indicates coverage for normal medical care throughout a woman's pregnancy, and sometimes it refers to the plan coverage for time spent in the hospital before and after giving birth. For this survey, we define maternity care as the medical coverage received throughout a woman's pregnancy, which usually includes diagnostic testing such as ultrasounds and fetal monitor procedures. Maternity care encompasses three stages: prenatal care, delivery care, and postnatal care.

When there were differences in coverage, report provisions for prenatal care. Physician office visits alone cannot be used as a proxy.

Synonyms: Maternity service, pregnancy care, maternity, or prenatal care.

Data Analysis Instructions

If the plan breaks out coverage details separately for office visits during the course of a woman's pregnancy versus childbirth, code for the office visits.

Instructions on Separate Limits

Report the dollar amount of copayments per visit. All other separate limits should be described in Remarks.

If the plan covers the stages of maternity care differently, code only the limits that apply to the portion of maternity care that does not take place in the hospital.

If maternity care coverage varies by primary care physicians versus specialists, report the provisions for specialists.

In some plans, the maternity care copayment only applies to the first visit, with the rest of the visits over the course of the woman's pregnancy covered with no copayment. In other cases, the maternity care copayment applies once to the entire pregnancy. In both of these cases, report the one-time nature of the copayment.

Example: A plan describes coverage for "hospital maternity care for mother and newborn" as having the same limits as hospital inpatient care. The same plan also indicates that "prenatal care" is covered with a $20 copayment.

Action: Report the $20 copayment because prenatal care aligns with the definition of maternity care we are using for this survey.

Infertility Treatment

Definition

Infertility treatment is defined as the services to diagnose and treat the causes of infertility. Some plans explicitly exclude coverage for advanced reproductive treatments such as in-vitro fertilization. Those same plans may also cover other infertility treatments, for which analysts should still report the limits.

Though infertility diagnosis is usually combined with the category of infertility services, in order to say that this benefit is covered, the plan must include some mention of treatment. If diagnosis is covered, but treatment is not, analysts should code that infertility treatment is excluded. Infertility treatment as defined above differs from family planning services, which usually encompass counseling, consultations, contraceptives, and sterilization.

Synonyms: Infertility treatment may also be called infertility services. Some of the specific infertility treatment services mentioned might include artificial insemination, ovulation induction, in-vitro fertilization, and other "advanced reproductive technology." Report for infertility treatment if the plan mentions "infertility treatment" in general or if at least one of the above listed services is mentioned.

Instructions on Separate Limits

In contrast to other benefits, report separate coinsurance limits for this benefit in the coinsurance answer box. All other separate limits should be described in Remarks.

If coverage for infertility services varies by location, report the provisions for outpatient settings and describe the limits for other settings in Remarks.

Example: The plan states that infertility treatment is covered at 50 percent in contrast to the overall plan coinsurance of 80 percent.

Action: This different coinsurance rate constitutes a separate limit. Report the 50 percent rate in the coinsurance rate box.

Sterilization

Definition

This benefit is defined as a surgical procedure for men or women to prevent future pregnancies.

Synonyms: The term sterilization is used most frequently, but the terms vasectomy (for men) and tubal ligation (for women) are also seen.

Data Analysis Instructions

It is common to see sterilization coverage in a plan with sterilization reversal coverage excluded. Analysts should not report for sterilization reversals.

Instructions on Separate Limits

Analysts will report for whether there are any separate limits for sterilization, but will not be prompted to enter a specific copayment. However, all separate limits should be described in Remarks.

Example: In the plan document, sterilization is listed as covered, but no details are given. However, office visits are covered in full after a $30 copayment, and surgery is covered at 100 percent at inpatient and outpatient facilities.

Action: Record that sterilization is "covered," but that coverage details are not mentioned in plan documents. We do not want to assume that sterilization is included under the more general term of surgical services or office visits. Specific limits for sterilization must be mentioned.

Gynecological Exams and Services

Definition

Gynecological exams are defined as the routine exam, not any associated tests (such as sonograms) that may result from the exam and not any non-routine exam such as a colposcopy or cervical biopsy. However, to be reported as a benefit, the plan must refer specifically to gynecological exams or one of the synonyms listed. Do not report annual physical exams as gynecological exams.

Synonyms: Gynecological visit, Pap smear, Papanicolaou (PAP) test, routine GYN Care, gynecological care exam, pelvic exam, or well woman exam. Plan language such as "OB/GYN," "OB/GYN visit," or "GYN visit" should be reported as indicating coverage of gynecological exams.

Instructions on Separate Limits

Report dollar copayments. All other separate limits should be described in Remarks.

If the plan mentions gynecological exams separate from Pap smear screenings, code for the exams limits rather than the limits for any associated tests. If the plan only mentions Pap smear limits, then code those limits for gynecological exam.

If the copayment varies by primary care physician (PCP)/doctor office visits and OB/GYN/specialists visits, code for the OB/GYN/specialist. This deviates from the rule of coding for the most generous item, but since specialists are more commonly used for gynecological exams, this is what is to be recorded.
Gynecologist exams may also be subject to an annual wellness benefit maximum and can be limited to one exam per year. Consider a limit of one exam per year as a separate limit.

Example: A plan describes coverage for "Pap smear screening" as being fully covered once a year. The same plan also indicates that "gynecological exam" is covered with a $15 copayment per PCP visit and a $30 copayment per specialist visit.

Action: Code for the $30 specialist visit copayment.

Example: The plan document mentions routine annual adult physical exams but does not mention that gynecological exams are covered. It also mentions "wellness."

Action: Do not code as a gynecological exam. There must be explicit mention of gynecological exams to be coded as such.

Organ and Tissue Transplantation

Definition

This benefit, sometimes called organ and tissue transplants, is the process by which human organs are surgically transferred from a donor to a recipient. Analysts of this benefit should only look at the coverage provided to the recipient and not at any benefits a donor may receive. Analysts also should focus on coverage provided for the surgical procedure and ignore any additional organ and tissue transplantation benefits that may be mentioned in the plan document such as coverage for travel and lodging.

Occasionally plans will mention specifically what organs are covered under the benefit.

- If the plan document does this, make sure that coverage is provided for the transplantation of the kidney, liver, heart or other major organs.
- If the plan lists out the organs that are covered for transplantation services and the above organs are not covered, report this benefit as excluded.
- If the plan only mentions transplantation services and says nothing about what organs are covered, report that the benefit is covered.

Synonyms: Human organ transplants, organ transplant benefits, transplantation services.

Instructions on Separate Limits

Analysts will report for whether there are any separate limits for organ and tissue transplantation services, but they will not be prompted to enter a specific copayment. However, all separate limits should be described in Remarks.

Frequently, organ and tissue transplantation is covered by overall limits of deductible and coinsurance. Sometimes there is an additional copayment or premium required for organ and tissue transplantation. The copayment could be described as either an organ and tissue transplantation copayment or as a physician copayment.

Ignore any hospital admission charges that may occur for organ and tissue transplantation. The analyst should note the existence of a separate limit.

Standard Errors

Estimates of standard errors are provided in this section for all the estimates of the 12 additional benefits, shown in tables 4 though 15. For ease of reference, the estimates of standard errors are presented in the same table formats and they are numbered accordingly, for example, the standard error table for data table 4 is table 4-S. Standard errors for tables 1 through 3 can be found in the publication *National Compensation Survey: Health Plan Provisions in Private Industry in the United States, 2008*, available online at http://www.bls.gov/ncs/ebs/detailedprovisions/2008/ebbl0042.pdf.

Standard errors are presented in percentages for the percentage estimates of participants by specific plan coverage details and for the estimates of separate coinsurance percentage rates for infertility treatment. Standard errors are presented in dollars for estimates of dollar copayment amounts.

NCS estimates are derived from a sample of occupations selected from the responding establishments. Two types of errors are possible in an estimate based on a sample survey: sampling errors and nonsampling errors. *Sampling errors* occur because the sample makes up only a part of the population. The sample used for the survey is one of a number of possible samples that could have been selected under the sample design, each producing its own estimate. A measure of the variation among sample estimates is the *standard error*. *Nonsampling errors* are data errors that stem from any source other than sampling error, such as data collection errors and data-processing errors.

Standard errors can be used to measure the precision with which an estimate from a particular sample approximates the expected result of all possible samples. The chances are about 68 out of 100 that an estimate from the survey differs from a complete population figure by less than the standard error. The chances are about 90 out of 100 that this difference would be less than 1.6 times the standard error. Statements of comparison based upon the tabular data appearing in these findings are significant at a level of 1.6 standard errors or better. This means that, for differences cited, the estimated difference is greater than 1.6 times the standard error of the difference. For details on how standard errors are calculated, see Chapter 8 of the *BLS Handbook of Methods* at: http://www.bls.gov/opub/hom/pdf/homch8.pdf.

Table 4-S. Standard Errors for Emergency Room Visits: Type of coverage, private industry workers, National Compensation Survey, 2009

Benefit coverage	All plans	Fee-for-service	Health maintenance organizations
Existence of Coverage			
With coverage	0.8	1.0	1.5
Without coverage	–	–	–
Not mentioned in plan documents	0.8	1.0	1.5
Extent of Coverage			
Covered in full	0.2	–	–
Subject to limits	0.9	1.0	1.5
Not mentioned in plan documents	0.3	–	–
Limits on Coverage			
Subject to plan limits	1.0	1.1	2.8
Subject to separate limits	1.3	1.4	1.6
With a copayment per visit	1.3	1.5	1.6
Copayment at 10th percentile	0	0	0
Copayment at 25th percentile	$17.66	$16.79	0
Copayment at 50th percentile (median)	0	0	0
Copayment at 75th percentile	0	0	$8.50
Copayment at 90th percentile	0	0	0
Not mentioned in plan documents	–	–	–

NOTE: Dashes indicate that no data were reported or that data do not meet publication criteria. For definitions of terms, see the Technical Note of this report.

Table 5-S. Standard Errors for Ambulance Services: Type of coverage, private industry workers, National Compensation Survey, 2009

Benefit coverage	All plans	Fee-for-service	Health maintenance organizations
Existence of Coverage			
With coverage	1.3	1.6	2.9
Without coverage	–	–	–
Not mentioned in plan documents	1.3	1.6	2.9
Extent of Coverage			
Covered in full	0.8	0.8	–
Subject to limits	1.4	1.6	3.3
Not mentioned in plan documents	0.4	0.4	–
Limits on Coverage			
Subject to plan limits	1.3	1.5	3.4
Subject to separate limits	1.2	1.1	3.5
Not mentioned in plan documents	0.3	0.4	–

NOTE: Dashes indicate that no data were reported or that data do not meet publication criteria. For definitions of terms, see the Technical Note of this report.

Table 6-S. Standard Errors for Diabetes Care Management: Type of coverage, private industry workers, National Compensation Survey, 2009

Benefit coverage	All plans	Fee-for-service	Health maintenance organizations
Existence of Coverage			
With coverage	1.2	1.4	2.1
Without coverage	–	–	–
Not mentioned in plan documents	1.2	1.4	2.1

NOTE: Dashes indicate that no data were reported or that data do not meet publication criteria. For definitions of terms, see the Technical Note of this report.

Table 7-S. Standard Errors for Kidney Dialysis: Type of coverage, private industry workers, National Compensation Survey, 2009

Benefit coverage	All plans	Fee-for-service	Health maintenance organizations
Existence of Coverage			
With coverage	1.3	1.6	1.8
Without coverage	–	–	–
Not mentioned in plan documents	1.3	1.6	1.8

NOTE: Dashes indicate that no data were reported or that data do not meet publication criteria. For definitions of terms, see the Technical Note of this report.

Table 8-S. Standard Errors for Physical Therapy: Type of coverage, private industry workers, National Compensation Survey, 2009

Benefit coverage	All plans	Fee-for-service	Health maintenance organizations
Existence of Coverage			
With coverage	1.3	1.6	2.4
Without coverage	–	–	–
Not mentioned in plan documents	1.3	1.6	2.4
Extent of Coverage			
Covered in full	–	–	–
Subject to limits	1.4	1.6	2.6
Not mentioned in plan documents	–	–	–
Limits on Coverage			
Subject to plan limits	1.3	1.5	3.3
Subject to separate limits	1.3	1.5	2.5
With a copayment per visit	1.3	1.2	3.1
Copayment at 10th percentile	$2.22	$6.27	0
Copayment at 25th percentile	$2.77	$4.16	0
Copayment at 50th percentile (median)	0	$0.20	$5.19
Copayment at 75th percentile	0	$5.89	0
Copayment at 90th percentile	$1.70	$0.98	0
Not mentioned in plan documents	–	0.2	–

NOTE: Dashes indicate that no data were reported or that data do not meet publication criteria. For definitions of terms, see the Technical Note of this report.

Table 9-S. Standard Errors for Durable Medical Equipment: Type of coverage, private industry workers, National Compensation Survey, 2009

Benefit coverage	All plans	Fee-for-service	Health maintenance organizations
Existence of Coverage			
With coverage	1.5	1.7	2.5
Without coverage	–	–	–
Not mentioned in plan documents	1.5	1.7	2.6
Extent of Coverage			
Covered in full	0.5	0.5	–
Subject to limits	1.5	1.8	2.5
Not mentioned in plan documents	0.6	0.5	–
Limits on Coverage			
Subject to plan limits	1.4	1.7	2.6
Subject to separate limits	1.3	1.4	2.8
Not mentioned in plan documents	0.5	0.6	–

NOTE: Dashes indicate that no data were reported or that data do not meet publication criteria. For definitions of terms, see the Technical Note of this report.

Table 10-S. Standard Errors for Prosthetics: Type of coverage, private industry workers, National Compensation Survey, 2009

Benefit coverage	All plans	Fee-for-service	Health maintenance organizations
Existence of Coverage			
With coverage	1.5	1.7	2.5
Without coverage	–	–	–
Not mentioned in plan documents	1.5	1.7	2.4
Extent of Coverage			
Covered in full	0.7	–	–
Subject to limits	1.5	1.7	2.2
Not mentioned in plan documents	0.5	–	–
Limits on Coverage			
Subject to plan limits	1.5	1.7	1.8
Subject to separate limits	0.9	1.0	2.2
Not mentioned in plan documents	0.4	0.6	–

NOTE: Dashes indicate that no data were reported or that data do not meet publication criteria. For definitions of terms, see the Technical Note of this report.

Table 11-S. Standard Errors for Maternity Care: Type of coverage, private industry workers, National Compensation Survey, 2009

Benefit coverage	All plans	Fee-for-service	Health maintenance organizations
Existence of Coverage			
With coverage	1.5	1.7	2.7
Without coverage	–	–	–
Not mentioned in plan documents	1.5	1.7	2.7
Extent of Coverage			
Covered in full	0.8	0.7	2.6
Subject to limits	1.4	1.8	2.9
Not mentioned in plan documents	0.4	0.5	0.3
Limits on Coverage			
Subject to plan limits	1.3	1.5	2.8
Subject to separate limits	1.3	1.5	3.0
With a copayment per visit	1.2	1.4	2.7
Copayment at 10th percentile	$4.77	0	0
Copayment at 25th percentile	0	$3.54	$5.56
Copayment at 50th percentile (median)	0	$3.68	0
Copayment at 75th percentile	0	0	$5.10
Copayment at 90th percentile	0	0	$2.60
Not mentioned in plan documents	0.4	0.4	–

NOTE: Dashes indicate that no data were reported or that data do not meet publication criteria. For definitions of terms, see the Technical Note of this report.

Table 12-S. Standard Errors for Infertility Treatment: Type of coverage, private industry workers, National Compensation Survey, 2009

Benefit coverage	All plans	Fee-for-service	Health maintenance organizations
Existence of Coverage			
With coverage	1.5	1.8	2.3
W ithout coverage	1.1	1.3	2.5
N ot mentioned in plan documents	1.7	2.2	2.8
Extent of Coverage			
C overed in full	0.1	–	0.1
S ubject to limits	1.5	1.8	2.3
N ot mentioned in plan documents	0.2	–	0.3
Limits on Coverage			
S ubject to plan limits	1.1	1.3	2.5
Subject to separate limits	1.3	1.4	2.3
With a copayment per visit	0.7	0.4	2.3
Coinsurance at 10th percentile	0	0	0
Coinsurance at 25th percentile	0	0	0
Coinsurance at 50th percentile (median)	0	7.8	0
Coinsurance at 75th percentile	17.5	16.1	0
Coinsurance at 90th percentile	10.0	0	23.9
N ot mentioned in plan documents	0.2	0.2	–

NOTE: Dashes indicate that no data were reported or that data do not meet publication criteria. For definitions of terms, see the Technical Note of this report.

Table 13-S. Standard Errors for Sterilization: Type of coverage, private industry workers, National Compensation Survey, 2009

Benefit coverage	All plans	Fee-for-service	Health maintenance organizations
Existence of Coverage			
With coverage	1.2	1.5	1.8
W ithout coverage	0.3	0.4	0.3
N ot mentioned in plan documents	1.3	1.6	1.8

NOTE: For definitions of terms, see the Technical Note of this report.

Table 14-S. Standard Errors for Gynecological Exams and Services: Type of coverage, private industry workers, National Compensation Survey, 2009

Benefit coverage	All plans	Fee-for-service	Health maintenance organizations
Existence of Coverage			
With coverage	1.4	1.6	3.4
W ithout coverage	–	–	–
N ot mentioned in plan documents	1.4	1.6	3.4
Extent of Coverage			
C overed in full	–	–	–
S ubject to limits	1.4	1.6	3.1
N ot mentioned in plan documents	–	–	–
Limits on Coverage			
S ubject to plan limits	1.3	1.5	3.0
Subject to separate limits	1.3	1.5	3.1
With a copayment per visit	1.2	1.4	2.7
Copayment at 10th percentile	0	–	0
Copayment at 25th percentile	0	–	0
Copayment at 50th percentile (median)	0	–	0
Copayment at 75th percentile	0	–	$5.00
Copayment at 90th percentile	$5.55	–	0
N ot mentioned in plan documents	–	–	–

NOTE: Dashes indicate that no data were reported or that data do not meet publication criteria. For definitions of terms, see the Technical Note of this report.

Table 15-S. Standard Errors for Organ and Tissue Transplantation: Type of coverage, private industry workers, National Compensation Survey, 2009

Benefit coverage	All plans	Fee-for-service	Health maintenance organizations
Existence of Coverage			
With coverage	1.6	2.1	2.5
W ithout coverage	–	–	–
N ot mentioned in plan documents	1.6	2.1	2.5
Extent of Coverage			
C overed in full	0.8	–	1.4
S ubject to limits	1.5	1.7	2.0
N ot mentioned in plan documents	0.3	–	1.1
Limits on Coverage			
S ubject to plan limits	1.5	1.8	1.9
Subject to separate limits	1.2	1.4	1.6
N ot mentioned in plan documents	0.6	0.7	–

NOTE: Dashes indicate that no data were reported or that data do not meet publication criteria. For definitions of terms, see the Technical Note of this report.